Dairy Free Book

A Women's 2-Week Step-by-Step Guide to a Dairy Free Diet, With Curated Recipes and a Sample Meal Plan

mf

Disclaimer

By reading this disclaimer, you are accepting the terms of the disclaimer in full. If you disagree with this disclaimer, please do not read the guide.

All of the content within this guide is provided for informational and educational purposes only, and should not be accepted as independent medical or other professional advice. The author is not a doctor, physician, nurse, mental health provider, or registered nutritionist/dietician. Therefore, using and reading this guide does not establish any form of a physician-patient relationship.

Always consult with a physician or another qualified health provider with any issues or questions you might have regarding any sort of medical condition. Do not ever disregard any qualified professional medical advice or delay seeking that advice because of anything you have read in this guide. The information in this guide is not intended to be any sort of medical advice and should not be used in lieu of any medical advice by a licensed and qualified medical professional.

The information in this guide has been compiled from a variety of known sources. However, the author cannot attest to or guarantee the accuracy of each source and thus should not be held liable for any errors or omissions.

You acknowledge that the publisher of this guide will not be held liable for any loss or damage of any kind incurred as a result of this guide or the reliance on any information provided within this guide. You acknowledge and agree that you assume all risk and responsibility for any action you undertake in response to the information in this guide.

Using this guide does not guarantee any particular result (e.g., weight loss or a cure). By reading this guide, you acknowledge that there are no guarantees to any specific outcome or results you can expect.

All product names, diet plans, or names used in this guide are for identification purposes only and are the property of their respective owners. The use of these names does not imply endorsement. All other trademarks cited herein are the property of their respective owners.

Where applicable, this guide is not intended to be a substitute for the original work of this diet plan and is, at most, a supplement to the original work for this diet plan and never a direct substitute. This guide is a personal expression of the facts of that diet plan.

Where applicable, persons shown in the cover images are stock photography models and the publisher has obtained the rights to use the images through license agreements with third-party stock image companies.

Table of Contents

Introduction

The majority, if not everyone, most likely believe that dairy products, the most well-known of which is milk, are great sources for various nutrients, particularly protein and calcium. Of course, they are not wrong. However, it is wrong to assume that dairy products and dairy-derived ingredients are not bad for your health.

Around 65% of the world's population is lactose intolerant, meaning they cannot consume most dairy products that contain lactose. There are also several people, mostly children, who are allergic to cow's milk. Moreover, even if you don't have these conditions, it still won't hurt to know how dairy and dairy derivatives may be bad for you in the long run.

In this guide, you'll learn about the following:
What a dairy-free diet is
How it can be beneficial to you
Types of food to avoid and consume
Sample meal plans to kick-start the diet program

If you decide to try out this dairy-free diet program, it's necessary that you take precautionary measures first before jumping right in. It's not easy and advisable to just change your eating habits. Like any diet plan, the goal is to achieve the healthiest version of yourself—be it to reduce weight, have a firmer body, or avoid illnesses. As a safety measure, you need to, first and foremost, seek medical and professional advice. This is because by going through this diet, you might experience changes in your body that may either be beneficial or harmful to your health.

Moving forward, the success of this diet plan will rely heavily on your self-discipline. Be consistent with your decision. This is for your health and wellness after all.

Chapter 1: What Is a Dairy-Free Diet?

A dairy-free diet is a meal plan that excludes all forms of dairy products, specifically foods that contain lactose, a disaccharide sugar, or a form of carbohydrates naturally present in dairy and milk. To not fully miss out on the nutrients found in dairy, this type of diet provides healthier alternatives and options to replace dairy products.

Before we get started, let's understand some basic background about dairy. Dairy products have been consumed by humans for thousands of years, providing essential nutrients such as calcium, protein, and vitamins. Historically, dairy was consumed for its health benefits, but it has also become a part of many cultural and culinary traditions. From milk to cheese to yogurt, dairy is a diverse and complex food group with a long history and a complex composition.

At its most basic level, dairy refers to products that are derived from the milk of cows, sheep, goats, or other mammals. Milk is composed of a variety of components, including water, proteins, carbohydrates, fats, vitamins, and minerals. The composition of milk can vary depending on the species of the mammal, the animal's diet, and other factors.

For example, cow's milk contains a different composition of proteins and fats than goat's milk.

One of the key components of milk is protein. Milk contains two main types of protein: casein and whey. Casein makes up about 80% of the protein in milk, while whey makes up the remaining 20%. Casein is a slow-digesting protein that provides a constant supply of amino acids to the body, while whey is a fast-digesting protein that is quickly absorbed by the body. This makes dairy an important source of protein for many people, particularly athletes and bodybuilders.

Another important component of dairy is calcium. Calcium is essential for strong bones and teeth, and dairy is one of the best sources of this nutrient. In fact, one cup of milk contains around 30% of the recommended daily intake of calcium. Cheese, yogurt, and other dairy products are also good sources of calcium.

In addition to protein and calcium, dairy also contains other important nutrients. For example, milk is a good source of vitamin D, which is important for bone health. It also contains vitamin B12, which is necessary for nerve function and DNA synthesis. Dairy products also contain minerals like potassium, magnesium, and zinc.

While dairy products are a good source of essential nutrients, they can also be high in fat and calories. Whole milk, cheese, and other full-fat dairy products can be particularly high in saturated fat, which can contribute to heart disease and other health problems. As a result, many people choose to consume low-fat or fat-free dairy products.

In addition to its nutritional composition, dairy has a long history and cultural significance. For example, dairy is an important part of many traditional cuisines, from French cheese to Indian lassi. Dairy products are also an important part of many religious and cultural traditions. For example, dairy products are often consumed during the Jewish holiday of Shavuot, while dairy is an important component of the Indian festival of Holi.

Dairy production and consumption has also had a significant impact on the environment. Dairy cows require large amounts of feed and water, and they produce significant amounts of waste. Large-scale dairy production can contribute to environmental problems such as water pollution, soil degradation, and greenhouse gas emissions.

In recent years, there has been increased interest in plant-based alternatives to dairy products. These products, which are often made from soy, almonds, or other plant-based sources, are marketed as a healthier and more sustainable alternative to dairy. While these products may offer some benefits, they may also have their own nutritional and environmental concerns.

In conclusion, dairy is a diverse and complex food group with a long history and significant cultural and nutritional significance. From milk to cheese to yogurt, dairy provides essential nutrients such as calcium and protein, but it can also be high in fat and calories.

As consumers become more conscious of their health and the environment, there is likely to be continued interest in both traditional dairy products and plant-based alternatives. Ultimately, the composition and impact of dairy production and consumption will continue to be an important area of study for scientists, policymakers, and consumers alike.

For some, it may be considered a challenge to fully exclude dairy products in their diet for various reasons. The question lies though, why do some people choose a dairy-free diet?

Experts say that the reasons for this have something to do with health and ethical concerns. For some, they choose to not consume dairy because of personal reasons such as culture and preference.

Health Concerns

Dairy is a good source of essential nutrients needed by the body, such as calcium, vitamins A, B12, and D, and protein, to name some. However, it is important to note that there are people who choose to refrain from consuming dairy because of various health reasons.

Probably the biggest in terms of numbers are those who are lactose intolerant or people who are unable to digest lactose. Lactose intolerance happens when a person does not have enough lactase enzyme to break down lactose, which is a form of carbohydrates in dairy products. Just in Asian countries alone, up to 80% of the population[1] experience this condition. Worldwide, around 65% of the population[2] is considered lactose intolerant.

---

[1] https://vegan.com/info/dairy-free/
[2] https://www.ncbi.nlm.nih.gov/books/NBK532285/

This digestive disorder may begin at birth or childhood, but it's typically rare. Usually, being lactose intolerant happens with age, as the body loses the ability to digest lactose. Another reason to end up experiencing this disorder is by an illness, either caused by a stomach bug or being diagnosed with a more serious illness that is celiac disease.

Lactose intolerance isn't exactly harmful, but it causes discomforts like diarrhea, bloatedness, gas, vomiting, nausea, constipation, and abdominal cramps.

For some, their reason for avoiding dairy is because of the fats that are present in most of them, like the highly saturated fat present in whole milk.

Another reason for some to avoid dairy products is allergies. Some people are allergic to protein present in milk, particularly infants and children. While the majority outgrows this, there are still some who experience adverse reactions towards dairy.

Some follow a dairy-free diet by choice because they benefited from the absence of dairy in their diet. Their symptoms have greatly improved, including digestive problems, nasal congestion, chronic ear infection, and acne.

Several studies on dairy consumption and its health effects are usually varied and have conflicting findings. This is important to note when researching the benefits of consuming or avoiding dairy in your diet.

Ethical Concerns

In terms of ethical practices, some oppose the industry that supplies dairy and veal products because of how these are acquired. By not consuming dairy products, they bring attention to the unethical treatment of animals that supply these products. Firstly, cattle are kept in cramped indoor spaces and not allowed to graze the grass. Secondly, young cattle are usually preferred to produce milk, as older ones don't produce as much anymore. These young cattle are made to get pregnant annually to harvest their milk. Thirdly, two-day-old calves are taken away from their mothers, as male calves commonly supply veal.

The people who question these practices point out that the high demand for dairy products gears the production of veal. If people would consider going dairy-free, it might help lessen or curb the need for harvesting veal from newborn calves.

Advantages and Disadvantages

Dairy products have been a staple in the human diet for thousands of years. Many people rely on dairy for its high calcium content and protein levels. However, the consumption of dairy also comes with potential advantages and disadvantages.

One main advantage of dairy consumption is the high calcium content found in milk, cheese, and yogurt. Calcium is essential for strong bones and teeth, and it is crucial for muscle function, nerve transmission, and blood clotting.

Dairy is one of the most significant dietary sources of calcium, making it an essential source of nutrients for children and adults.

Moreover, the protein found in dairy products is a complete source of essential amino acids, making it a perfect protein source for those looking to build muscle, maintain lean tissue, and support healthy growth.

Dairy products also contain an array of other essential vitamins and minerals, including vitamin D, which is necessary for healthy bones and teeth, vitamin B12, which is essential for the nervous system and red blood cell production, and potassium, which helps regulate blood pressure.

However, dairy consumption also comes with potential disadvantages. One significant disadvantage is the lactose found in dairy products, which can cause digestive issues in those with lactose intolerance. Lactose intolerance affects around 65% of the world's population, and it occurs when the body is unable to digest lactose properly due to a shortage of the enzyme lactase.

Another potential disadvantage of dairy comes from the fat content found in many of its products. High-fat dairy products like cheese and butter can be a significant source of saturated fat, which can raise cholesterol levels and increase the risk of heart disease. Additionally, many dairy products are high in calories, which can cause weight gain if consumed in excess.

Despite the advantages and disadvantages of dairy consumption, it is essential to seek professional health advice before making any dietary changes. A qualified healthcare professional can provide insight into the best diet for an individual's specific needs and goals while taking into consideration any potential health concerns or dietary restrictions.

Differences between Lactose-Free and Dairy-Free
To be clear, lactose-free and dairy-free aren't the same. When a product states it's dairy-free, it means that that product doesn't contain milk or milk-derived ingredients.[3] A lactose-free product means it doesn't contain naturally occurring sugar or lactose. There are dairy products that contain less lactose and aid in digestion such as yogurt and some cheeses.[4] People who are allergic to milk need to stay away from lactose-free products and strictly stick to dairy-free products. On the other hand, lactose-free people may still reap the benefits of consuming dairy-free products.[5]

---

[3] https://www.eatthis.com/lactose-free-vs-dairy-free-difference/
[4] https://www.hsph.harvard.edu/nutritionsource/dairy/#:~:text=Bottom%20 Line,that%20 may%20 benefit%20 digestive%20health
[5] https://www.eatthis.com/lactose-free-vs-dairy-free-difference/

Chapter 2: Dairy-Free Diet: Foods to Avoid

Taking up a dairy-free diet plan means that you are going to exclude food that contains milk or ingredients that have milk in them. If you're thinking of ice cream, yogurt, cheese, and the likes, you might have to start saying goodbye to them.

The examples listed above are just a few of the things you need to start removing from your diet. There are a lot of food products that contain dairy or modified dairy ingredients. It's highly recommended that you learn how to read the back labels and identify the dairy ingredients, some of which are such as butter flavored, whey, whey butter, whey cream caseinates, casein, lactose, hydrolysates, lactalbumin, and many more.

Here are some examples of products that may contain dairy ingredients:

Processed meats
Sliced ham, hotdogs, prosciutto, and other processed meat products can contain modified milk ingredients, which serve as fillers so there won't be a need to use up too much meat.

Canned tuna
Casein, which is a modified milk ingredient, can be found in canned tuna.

Vinaigrette salad dressing

Some vinaigrette salad dressings contain cheese for flavor and texture enhancement.

Tomato sauce

Some manufacturers produce canned tomato sauces that are embedded with cheese flavors. Some are even labeled as original or made from fresh tomatoes. However, the back label may tell you otherwise.

Flavored potato chips

Cheese-flavored chips will no doubt top this kind, but even the other flavored chips like barbecue and ketchup may contain dairy-derived ingredients.

Bread

Some types of bread include skim milk powders, butter, and whey powder as ingredients. However, do take note that there is also bread free from modified dairy ingredients.

Chewing gum

Chewing gums must also be avoided when following a strict dairy-free diet. Some manufacturers include milk proteins in producing chewing gums.

Protein powder

Lots of protein powders have dairy ingredients like whey. However, there are dairy-free protein powders, especially for vegans.

Coffee creamers

Casein can be found in creamers. There are lactose-free creamers available in the market, but there's no guarantee that these don't contain dairy ingredients.

Prepackaged seasoned rice
By nature, rice does not have any dairy component. However, that usually isn't the case anymore when it's mixed with other flavors. For example, butter, a dairy product, keeps the rice grains from sticking together.

Margarine
Margarine is widely known to be dairy-free because it is different from butter. However, some types of margarine have modified dairy ingredients such as casein and whey.

Crackers
Dairy-derived ingredients are largely used in manufacturing crackers. It is primarily used to extend the lifespan of the products and to improve the products' textures.

Dark chocolate
Some might misunderstand that dark chocolate is entirely different from milk chocolate. It isn't. Dark chocolate still contains milk-derived ingredients to enhance its flavor and texture.

Cereals
Cereals are one of those food types that can be produced without using any dairy ingredients. However, there are a variety of cereals that are either free of dairy or not. The only way to differentiate them is by checking the labels.

Now that you have a list of foods you need to watch out for when starting the dairy-free diet, you can start curating the food you have in storage or your future grocery list. Familiarizing yourself with the different types of dairy products and dairy-derivative ingredients will be a great start in helping you identify other food types that you need to avoid while doing this diet.

Chapter 3: Dairy-Free Diet: Best Dairy Substitutes

It may seem overwhelming to learn that there are a lot of food types, even staples that need to go when you start doing your dairy-free diet. Don't be discouraged though, because there are products available in the market that serve as the best alternative non-dairy foods for your usual dairy choices. You will enjoy these foods included in the list.

Vegan milk

For those who love to drink milk, there's a vegan option for you. Vegan milk includes soy milk, rice milk, almond milk, hemp seed milk, and coconut milk. Vegan milk is as versatile as fresh milk, as it can be enjoyed with a bowl of cereal or poured into some mouth-watering dishes. Vegan milk is considered to be more cost-efficient, environment-friendly, and even better for your health as compared to the usual dairy milk.

Non-dairy yogurts

Yogurt is usually made by fermenting cow's milk. However, there is non-dairy yogurt, too. These are usually made out of soy milk and coconut milk, which are perfectly free from any dairy fats. Other dairy-free yogurts are made out of cashews, as well as a combination of pili nuts, coconuts, cassava, plantains, and lime.

Non-dairy cheese

Most non-dairy cheeses are made from solidified vegetable oils, soy protein, nuts like almonds and cashews, thickening agar flakes, vegetable glycerin, tapioca flour, bacterial cultures, arrowroots, and natural enzymes.

Vegan butter

Vegan butter is plant-based butter. These types of butter are commonly made from plant-based oils like avocado, olive, palm, kernel, and coconut. These oils or a combination of them are then mixed with water, emulsifiers, salt, natural and artificial flavors, and colorings to get the butter-like taste and texture.

Vegan butter is closer to margarine than real butter but is guaranteed dairy-free as compared to margarine.

Non-dairy ice cream

For die-hard ice cream lovers, here's a treat for you, there are ice cream substitutes available for you to enjoy. The best option is different fruit-flavored smoothies. There is also ice cream made from plant-based ingredients like soy, coconut, and almond milk.

Non-dairy sour creams

If you want to be certain of the ingredients, you can create your sour creams using tofu, cashews, or sunflower seeds. For convenience's sake, you can use plain non-dairy yogurt as a non-dairy sour cream alternative.

Non-dairy creams

Non-dairy creams contain fewer fats and calories than those that are dairy-based. These are commonly made of coconut milk. Plant-based creams do not have protein like any non-dairy alternatives, but they usually contain carbohydrates.

Chapter 4: Benefits of Dairy-Free Diet Plan for Women

Diet plans tailored to cut off dairy in your meals have proven to be beneficial not only for those who have digestive or allergy problems but even to those who want to either lose weight or get rid of acne problems. In this chapter, we'll focus on how beneficial this diet plan is for women.

Getting rid of acne

Women who follow the dairy-free diet plan swear by how it helped them get rid of acne breakout, as it is believed that consuming dairy contributes to this.

Research says there may be different reasons to support the previous statement. One is due to the milk produced by cows. Milking cows are injected with hormones that can increase the amount of milk a cow normally produces. This particular hormonal substance present in cow's milk is believed to cause an imbalance in women's hormones, which then results in acne breakouts.

Another possible cause is the growth hormones present in dairy products. One other possible cause is the highly refined ingredients and treated sugars added to dairy products. These additional ingredients can upset the normal insulin levels in the body, which will then trigger acne breakouts.

One dairy-free diet user shared her experience on how the diet program helped her get rid of her acne breakouts. Daley

Quinn had tried a lot of products in an attempt to get rid of her breakouts but nothing happened. That was until she tried the dairy-free diet program. She shared that she found the diet plan difficult and challenging at first, but she persisted. After three months of going dairy-free, she finally saw the effect of her perseverance by having acne-free skin.

Fertility

Another health benefit that a woman can get when doing a dairy-free diet is having a greater chance at ovulatory fertility.

A study conducted by Harvard faculty Jorge E. Chavarro, Janet W. Rich-Edwards, Bernard A. Rosner, and Walter C. Willet entitled "A prospective study of dairy foods intake and anovulatory infertility,"[6] suggested that ovulatory fertility can be impaired by dairy and lactose intakes.

To prove its validity, the research was done by monitoring the diet and condition of 18,555 women who are married and are in the premenopausal stage. These women do not have any infertility history. In the study, they attempted to get pregnant for a timetable of eight years.

In the study's conclusion, low-fat dairy products are one of the contributors to a woman's infertility. Moreover, fertility can be preserved when lactose is taken lightly or consumed just on a normal basis.

---

[6] https://pubmed.ncbi.nlm.nih.gov/17329264/

Another proof of dairy being a culprit for infertility is an experience shared by Alisa Vitti on a blog post. In her testimony, her dairy intakes had triggered her PCOS symptoms like acne, weight gain, and depression. She strongly suggested for her clients who are experiencing heavy periods, fibroids, PMS, or endometriosis to avoid dairy foods, even citing the following reasons on why they should do it:

1. Intestinal tracts can be inflamed by dairy components which will then result in some problems like irregular menstrual cycles or missing it. It can also interrupt ovulation and cause infertility.
2. Artificial growth hormones found in dairy foods can outdo estrogens.
3. Antibiotics found in dairy foods can interrupt estrogen metabolism. It can also badly affect the immune system.
4. Milking cows are fed with GMO soy and corn, which will cause an overload in estrogen count.
5. Adrenal and pituitary glands can be badly affected by dairy intakes through depleting magnesium reserves in your body.

These are just two of the benefits that one can get from following a dairy-free diet. Take note that it's important to note that a doctor's recommendation is still a must before starting this diet program.

Chapter 5: Dairy-Free Diet Meal Plan – Week One

There are a lot of benefits one can gain from going dairy-free, even for just a couple of weeks. Before starting the program, it's best to consult with your doctor or a licensed dietitian first, so you can go about the program safely and healthily.

For the first week, it's good to focus on slowly removing dairy products and dairy-derivative ingredients in your usual meals. This is to help you become more familiar with identifying these various dairy types and ingredients. In addition, you can also try to cook your usual meals but substitute dairy ingredients with dairy-free alternatives. Review the third chapter to get more familiar with dairy-free alternatives when preparing your usual meal.

It's also advisable that you keep a diary documenting your experiences as you start this diet program. This will help you keep track of the changes you experience in your body as you transition from your old lifestyle to a dairy-free lifestyle. It'll also be helpful for your doctor or dietitian to read about your experiences the next time you visit them again.

To get you started, here's a sample weekly plan featuring the easiest meals[7] to help you with the transition. The meals featured in this plan require ingredients that are most likely already in your pantry or are easy to find.

---

[7] https://www.godairyfree.org/news/easy-dairy-free-meal-plan

DAY	BREAKFAST	LUNCH	DINNER
1	Eggs, bacon, and dairy-free toast	Salad with dairy-free vinaigrette	Turkey or veggie burger
2	Granola or cereal with dairy-free or vegan milk	Salad sandwich	Dairy-free spaghetti
3	Fruit or dairy-free chocolate smoothie	Burrito wrap	Tacos with avocados
4	Oatmeal with nuts, dried fruits, or brown sugar	Chicken noodle soup	Kabobs
5	Dairy-free toast and fruit juice	Baked falafel	Black bean chili
6	Dairy-free pancakes with maple syrup or fresh fruits	BLT with avocado sandwich	Stir-fry veggies
7	Repeat any of your favorites	Pasta salad	Broiled or steamed fish with olive oil

Chapter 6: Dairy-Free Diet Meal Plan – Week Two

Now that you've experienced preparing usual meals minus the dairy and dairy derivatives, you're most likely ready to prepare new meals that are sure to add excitement to your diet program. If you see an improvement over the course of those two weeks, perhaps that may motivate you to adapt to the diet program for longer, even for a lifetime.

To get you started, here's a sample weekly plan for you. This may help you jumpstart your diet plan if you're still looking for ideas in case you want to eventually create your meal plans.

DAY	BREAKFAST	LUNCH	DINNER
Monday	Healthy baked oatmeal	Roasted veggies	Baked flounder
Tuesday	Toasted muesli	Spinach and watercress salad	Vegan pesto
Wednesday	Mango honey green smoothie	Mixed vegetable roast with lemon zest	Spinach and chickpeas
Thursday	Tofu scramble	Salmon, and asparagus	Zucchini, celery greens soup
Friday	Avocado egg toast	Arugula and mushroom salad	Tahini salmon
Saturday	Blueberry-banana overnight oats	Seafood stew	Tomato and basil soup
Sunday	Gala apple honeydew smoothie	Tomato clams	Cauliflower and mushrooms bake

Dairy-free Meal Recipes

You are now very close to living a dairy-free life anytime, soon! At this point, you can look at these delicious non-dairy recipes and try making them in the comfort of your home.

Healthy Baked Oatmeal

Ingredients:
- 2 cups rolled oats
- 1/2 cup almond milk
- 1/4 cup maple syrup
- 1/4 cup unsweetened applesauce
- 1 teaspoon vanilla extract
- 1/2 teaspoon cinnamon
- 1/4 teaspoon salt
- 1/4 cup chopped nuts (optional)
- 1/4 cup dried fruits (optional)

Instructions:
1. Preheat the oven to 350°F (175°C) and lightly grease a baking dish.
2. In a mixing bowl, combine the rolled oats, almond milk, maple syrup, applesauce, vanilla extract, cinnamon, and salt. Stir until well combined.
3. If desired, stir in the chopped nuts and dried fruits.
4. Pour the mixture into the prepared baking dish and spread it evenly.
5. Bake for 25-30 minutes or until the top is golden brown and the oatmeal is set.
6. Remove from the oven and let it cool for a few minutes before serving.

Creamy Tomato Soup

Ingredients:
- 1 can of crushed tomatoes
- 1 onion, chopped
- 2 garlic cloves, minced
- 1 tbsp of olive oil
- 1 cup of vegetable broth
- 1 cup of coconut milk
- Salt and pepper, to taste
- Basil leaves, chopped

Instructions:
1. In a large pot, heat the olive oil over medium heat.
2. Sauté the onions and garlic until they become translucent.
3. Add the crushed tomatoes, vegetable broth, and coconut milk. Stir to combine.
4. Bring the mixture to a boil and then reduce heat to a simmer.
5. Simmer for 15-20 minutes or until the soup has thickened.
6. Season with salt and pepper to taste.
7. Serve in bowls and garnish with basil leaves.

Chickpea Curry

Ingredients:
- 1 can of chickpeas, drained
- 1 onion, chopped
- 2 tbsp of olive oil
- 2 garlic cloves, minced
- 1 tbsp of curry powder
- 1 tsp of cumin powder
- 1 can of diced tomatoes
- 1 cup of vegetable broth
- Salt and pepper, to taste
- Cilantro leaves, chopped

Instructions:
1. In a large pot, heat the olive oil over medium heat.
2. Sauté the onions and garlic until they become translucent.
3. Add the curry powder and cumin powder. Stir to combine.
4. Add the chickpeas, diced tomatoes, and vegetable broth. Stir to combine.
5. Bring the mixture to a boil and then reduce heat to a simmer.
6. Simmer for 15-20 minutes or until the curry has thickened.
7. Season with salt and pepper to taste.
8. Serve in bowls and garnish with cilantro leaves.

Sweet Potato and Lentil Stew

Ingredients:
- 1 onion, chopped
- 2 garlic cloves, minced
- 1 tbsp of olive oil
- 2 sweet potatoes, peeled and cubed
- 1 cup of green lentils, rinsed
- 1 can of diced tomatoes
- 1 cup of vegetable broth
- 1 tsp of smoked paprika
- Salt and pepper, to taste
- Parsley leaves, chopped

Instructions:
1. In a large pot, heat the olive oil over medium heat.
2. Sauté the onions and garlic until they become translucent.
3. Add the sweet potatoes and green lentils. Stir to combine.
4. Add the diced tomatoes and vegetable broth. Stir to combine.
5. Add the smoked paprika, salt, and pepper. Stir to combine.
6. Bring the mixture to a boil and then reduce heat to a simmer.
7. Simmer for 30-35 minutes or until the sweet potatoes are tender and the lentils are fully cooked.
8. Serve in bowls and garnish with parsley leaves.

Quinoa Salad

Ingredients:
- 2 cups of cooked quinoa
- 1 can of black beans, drained and rinsed
- 1 red bell pepper, chopped
- 1 yellow bell pepper, chopped
- 1/2 red onion, chopped
- 1 avocado, diced
- 3 tbsp of olive oil
- 2 tbsp of lime juice
- Salt and pepper, to taste
- Cilantro leaves, chopped

Instructions:
1. In a large bowl, combine the cooked quinoa, black beans, red bell pepper, yellow bell pepper, red onion, and avocado.
2. In a small bowl, whisk together the olive oil, lime juice, salt, and pepper to make the dressing.
3. Pour the dressing over the quinoa mixture and toss to coat.
4. Serve in bowls and garnish with cilantro leaves.

Spinach Artichoke Dip

Ingredients:
- 1 cup raw cashews, soaked in hot water for 30 minutes
- 1 small clove garlic, minced
- 2 tablespoons nutritional yeast
- 1 tablespoon fresh lemon juice
- 1/2 teaspoon sea salt
- 1/2 teaspoon onion powder
- 1/4 teaspoon smoked paprika
- 1/4 teaspoon ground black pepper
- 1 cup frozen chopped spinach, thawed and squeezed dry
- 1 cup chopped artichoke hearts

Instructions:
1. Preheat the oven to 375°F.
2. Drain the soaked cashews and add them to a blender or food processor along with the minced garlic, nutritional yeast, lemon juice, sea salt, onion powder, smoked paprika, and black pepper. Blend until smooth.
3. Add the thawed and squeezed dry spinach and chopped artichoke hearts to the blender or food processor and pulse until mixed in but still chunky.
4. Transfer the spinach artichoke dip to an oven-safe baking dish and bake for 20-25 minutes, until heated through and bubbly on top. Serve hot with chips or veggies for dipping.

Roasted Cauliflower Soup

Ingredients:
- 1 head cauliflower, cut into florets
- 1 tablespoon olive oil
- 1/2 teaspoon sea salt
- 1/4 teaspoon ground black pepper
- 4 cups vegetable broth
- 1 large onion, diced
- 2 cloves garlic, minced
- 1 teaspoon ground cumin
- 1/2 teaspoon ground coriander
- 1/4 teaspoon smoked paprika
- 1/2 teaspoon dried thyme
- 1/2 teaspoon dried rosemary
- 1 bay leaf
- 1/4 cup chopped fresh parsley

Instructions:
1. Preheat the oven to 400°F. Toss the cauliflower florets with the olive oil, sea salt, and ground black pepper on a baking sheet. Roast in the oven for 25-30 minutes, until the cauliflower is tender and golden brown.
2. Heat a large pot over medium heat and add the diced onion. Sauté until the onion is soft and translucent, about 5-7 minutes. Add the minced garlic, ground cumin, ground coriander, smoked paprika, dried thyme, and dried rosemary to the pot. Stir to combine and cook for another 1-2 minutes, until fragrant.

3. Add the roasted cauliflower florets to the pot along with the vegetable broth and bay leaf. Bring everything to a boil, then reduce the heat to a simmer and cover the pot with a lid. Let cook for 20-25 minutes, until the cauliflower is very soft and easy to mash with a fork.

4. Remove the bay leaf from the pot and use an immersion blender or transfer the soup to a blender in batches and blend until smooth.

Conclusion

Dairy, while a valuable source of nutrients such as calcium, protein, and vitamin A, has been proven to be a type of food that can be replaced by better and healthier alternatives.

The need for these alternatives of course stems from those who have problems consuming dairy. Having this access to better substitutes, it's only right for us to take advantage of these better options to improve our health.

Following a dairy-free diet[8] will be challenging, but be assured that it'll be extremely worth it, especially for women looking into improving their lifestyles. Not only will it benefit our health, but also the environment and animal welfare.

So next time you're in the kitchen wondering what to cook for dinner, consider trying out some dairy-free recipes. You never know, you might just find a new favorite dish that not only tastes great, but is also better for your body and the planet.

So turn down the heat on that pot of mac and cheese and give these dairy-free options a chance!

---

[8]

References
https://vegan.com/info/dairy-free/
https://www.verywellfit.com/what-is-a-dairy-free-diet-1324040
https://worldpopulationreview.com/country-rankings/lactose-intolerance-by-country
https://vegan.com/info/dairy-free/
https://www.forkly.com/food/21-surprising-foods-to-avoid-on-a-dairy-free-diet/
https://www.webmd.com/diet/foods-high-in-lactose#
https://www.purewow.com/food/best-dairy-free-yogurt
https://www.eatthis.com/dairy-free-diet/
https://www.notsocheesykitchen.com/2017/07/what-is-non-dairy-cheese.html
https://www.healthline.com/nutrition/plant-butter
https://www.verywellfit.com/best-dairy-free-ice-creams-4694541
https://www.healthline.com/nutrition/dairy-substitutes#TOC_TITLE_HDR_8
https://www.healthline.com/health/dairy-and-acne#what-the-research-says
https://www.ovulifemd.com/dairy-and-fertility/
https://pubmed.ncbi.nlm.nih.gov/17329264/
https://www.thespruceeats.com/healthy-and-dairy-free-breakfasts-1001349
https://www.thespruceeats.com/healthy-vegan-baked-oatmeal-recipe-1001155
https://www.thespruceeats.com/toasted-muesli-recipe-256195
https://www.thespruceeats.com/mango-honey-green-smoothie-recipe-3377402
https://www.thespruceeats.com/tofu-scramble-with-salsa-3376578
https://www.eatingwell.com/recipe/267169/avocado-egg-toast/
https://www.eatingwell.com/recipe/268085/blueberry-banana-overnight-oats/
https://bit.ly/3vqs9DE
https://www.floliving.com/benefits-of-a-dairy-free-diet-for-women/
https://www.womenshealthmag.com/food/a21641590/cut-dairy-for-acne/